EVERYTHING ABOUT HODGKIN LYMPHOMA

A Complete Guide For Patients, Caregivers, And Healthcare Professionals - Causes, Symptoms, Diagnosis, Treatment, Coping Strategies, And More

DR. CADE JOSUE

Table of Contents

DISCLAIMER

The information provided in this book is for general informational purposes only. It is not intended as medical advice, diagnosis, or treatment.

The content of this book should not be considered a substitute for professional medical advice. Readers should consult with a qualified healthcare provider for diagnosis and treatment of any medical conditions they have.

While every effort has been made to ensure the accuracy and completeness of the information presented, the author makes no representations or warranties of any kind, express or implied, about the completeness, accuracy, reliability, suitability, or availability with respect to the information, contained in this book.

The author disclaims any responsibility for any loss or damage resulting from reliance on the information provided in this book. References to individuals, products, websites, organizations, or other names are for informational purposes only and do not imply endorsement.

By reading this book, readers acknowledge that they are responsible for their own health decisions and should seek appropriate medical advice when necessary.

<u>ABOUT THIS BOOK</u>

"Everything About Hodgkin Lymphoma" is an indispensable resource that offers exhaustive insights into numerous facets of the disease, catering to healthcare personnel as well as individuals affected by Hodgkin lymphoma. An introductory section initiates this book, establishing the foundation for an exhaustive examination of Hodgkin lymphoma.

"Understanding Hodgkin Lymphoma" provides a comprehensive analysis of the disease, shedding light on its epidemiology, pathophysiology, and other essential facets. The "Causes and Risk Factors" chapter provides an in-depth analysis of the elements that contribute to the onset of Hodgkin lymphoma, thereby facilitating more accurate risk evaluations and mitigation approaches.

The chapter titled "Signs and Symptoms" delineates the various presentations of Hodgkin lymphoma, thereby enabling timely identification and effective treatment. This book "Diagnostic Procedures" provides a comprehensive explanation of the diverse methodologies utilized in the diagnosis of Hodgkin lymphoma, guaranteeing precise evaluation and prompt initiation of treatment.

"Staging and Classification" provides clinicians with an understanding of the staging criteria and classification systems that are applied to Hodgkin lymphoma. This knowledge aids in the determination of prognosis and treatment approaches. "Treatment Options" provides an exhaustive synopsis of therapeutic approaches, encompassing supportive care measures, radiation therapy, immunotherapy, stem cell transplantation, targeted therapy, and chemotherapy.

Subsequent chapters provide comprehensive analyses of each treatment modality, elucidating their respective mechanisms, indications, efficacy, and potential adverse effects. Furthermore, this books "Prognosis and Survival Rates" provides significant contributions by shedding light on the enduring consequences of Hodgkin lymphoma, thereby assisting medical professionals and individuals afflicted with the disease in making well-informed choices concerning treatment and subsequent monitoring.

"Prevention Strategies" elucidates proactive measures that can be implemented by individuals to mitigate the likelihood of developing Hodgkin lymphoma. "Current Research and Advances" delves into burgeoning developments and novel approaches in the realm of Hodgkin lymphoma research, presenting a glimmer of optimism regarding prospective progress in the areas of diagnosis and treatment.

In conclusion, "Living with Hodgkin Lymphoma" examines the psychosocial dimensions of managing the illness, offering assistance and direction to individuals afflicted with the disease as well as their loved ones during this trying period. Fundamentally, "Everything About Hodgkin Lymphoma" functions as an all-encompassing compilation, furnishing healthcare professionals and patients with the requisite information to adeptly navigate the intricacies associated with Hodgkin lymphoma.

CHAPTER ONE

A Brief Overview Of Hodgkin Lymphoma

Hodgkin lymphoma (HL), alternatively referred to as Hodgkin's disease, is a malignancy that develops within the lymphatic system. It was given its name in 1832, the year Thomas Hodgkin first described it. Hémolytic lenticular (HL) is distinguished by the aberrant proliferation of Reed-Sternberg cells, a subtype of B lymphocytes.

Hodgkin lymphoma is an infrequent malignancy in comparison to other types of cancer, comprising an estimated 0.5% of the total cancer incidence in the United States.

Nevertheless, early diagnosis and treatment contribute significantly to its high survival rate, making it one of the most curable forms of cancer.

Comprehension Of Hodgkin Lymphoma

Although Hodgkin lymphoma can manifest at any stage of life, its incidence is highest among young adults aged 15 to 35 and elderly adults aged 55 and older at the time of diagnosis. Slightly more frequently observed in males than in females.

Two Primary Subtypes Of Hodgkin Lymphoma:

1. Classical Hodgkin Lymphoma (cHL) constitutes the prevailing subtype, comprising an estimated 95% of the total cases of HL. It is characterized by the presence of Reed-Sternberg cells, which are large, aberrant B lymphocytes. Classical Hodgkin lymphoma is additionally classified into subtypes according to the microscopic examination of Reed-Sternberg cells and other distinguishing features. Hodgkin lymphoma with mixed cellularity, lymphocyte-rich Hodgkin lymphoma,

lymphocyte-depleted Hodgkin lymphoma, and nodular sclerosis Hodgkin lymphoma are the subtypes.

2. Nodular lymphocyte-predominant Hodgkin lymphoma (NLPHL) constitutes an estimated 5% of the total HL cases. Classical Hodgkin lymphoma is distinguished from lymphocyte-predominant cells, which are massive, popcorn-like cells. These cells are distinct from Reed-Sternberg cells. Although the precise etiology of Hodgkin lymphoma remains unknown, it is hypothesized to arise from a complex interplay of genetic, environmental, and immune system influences. The following are risk factors for Hodgkin lymphoma:

Risk Factors And Causes

1. An elevated susceptibility to developing Hodgkin lymphoma or other lymphomas may be observed in individuals with a familial

predisposition to the condition. A minority of Hodgkin lymphoma cases may contain a genetic component, even though the disease is exceptionally rare.

2. Individuals who have a compromised immune system, including those who are taking immunosuppressive medications or who have HIV/AIDS or have undergone organ transplantation, are at an elevated risk of developing Hodgkin lymphoma.

3. Infection with the Epstein-Barr virus (EBV), the causative agent of infectious mononucleosis (mono), has been associated with an elevated propensity for developing Hodgkin lymphoma, specifically among the young adult population. Hodgkin lymphoma does not develop in the majority of individuals infected with EBV; this suggests that additional factors contribute to the progression of the disease.

4. The incidence of Hodgkin lymphoma is comparatively higher among young adults aged 15 to 35 and elderly adults aged 55 and above, irrespective of gender. Furthermore, there exists a marginally higher incidence of Hodgkin lymphoma in males compared to females.

5. Prior Cancer Treatment: Individuals with a medical history of Hodgkin lymphoma who have received specific forms of cancer treatment, including chemotherapy or radiation therapy, for other malignancies, may be at an elevated risk of developing the disease in the future.

6. Specific Viral Infections: Hodgkin lymphoma risk is elevated in individuals infected with human immunodeficiency virus (HIV) and human T-cell lymphotropic virus type 1 (HTLV-1), in addition to Epstein-Barr virus.

7. Further investigation is required to validate the assertions that specific chemical exposure,

including that associated with pesticides, solvents, and other environmental pollutants, could elevate the likelihood of developing Hodgkin lymphoma.

Overall, a combination of genetic predisposition, environmental factors, viral infections, and immune system dysfunction likely contribute to the development of Hodgkin lymphoma, although the precise cause of the disease remains uncertain. Recognizing these risk factors can facilitate the identification of individuals who are potentially more vulnerable and could benefit from heightened surveillance or preventative measures.

Symptoms And Indications

The manifestations and symptoms of Hodgkin lymphoma are subject to considerable individual variation and may be affected by the disease's size and scope. Frequent manifestations consist of:

1. Frequently, the most conspicuous manifestation is the enlargement of lymph nodes, which commonly occurs in the groin, armpits, or neck. While these enlarged lymph nodes are typically asymptomatic, any distress may result from their pressure on adjacent structures.

2. Weight loss that is both substantial and unexplained, frequently surpassing 10% of the individual's body weight, may manifest in patients diagnosed with Hodgkin lymphoma.

3. Fever and shivers: A prevalent manifestation of HL is persistent fever, which is frequently accompanied by shivers. Fever may manifest intermittently and devoid of a discernible etiology.

4. Prolonged perspiration, especially during the night, constitutes an additional hallmark manifestation of Hodgkin lymphoma. Severe night perspiration has the potential to disturb sleep patterns.

5. A significant number of patients with HL suffer from severe fatigue that cannot be alleviated by rest. The effects of this fatigue on daily activities and quality of life can be substantial.

6. Persistent Cough or Shortness of Breath: Chest-stage Hodgkin lymphoma may give rise to symptoms including chest pain, persistent wheezing, or respiratory distress.

7. Pruritus, which refers to the irritation of the skin, is an infrequent yet significant manifestation of HL. Although the precise etiology of pruritus in Hodgkin lymphoma remains unknown, it is hypothesized that specific substances secreted by the aberrant lymphocytes contribute to this condition. It is crucial to acknowledge that these symptoms may arise from factors unrelated to Hodgkin lymphoma. However, to obtain an accurate diagnosis, individuals who are experiencing persistent or concerning symptoms should seek medical evaluation.

CHAPTER TWO

Diagnostic Procedures

Hodgkin lymphoma is commonly identified through a comprehensive evaluation of the patient's medical records, physical assessment, and a battery of diagnostic examinations. Important diagnostic procedures and tests for HL include:

1. Physical Examination: A comprehensive physical examination is performed, paying specific attention to the lymph nodes, spleen, and other organs, to evaluate for indications of lymphoma.

2. Imaging Studies: To visualize the extent of lymphoma involvement in the body, imaging techniques such as computed tomography (CT), magnetic resonance imaging (MRI), and positron emission tomography (PET) scans are

utilized. These imaging modalities aid in the localization and quantification of impacted lymph nodes, as well as the identification of extra-organ involvement.

3. Biopsy: The definitive diagnostic procedure for Hodgkin lymphoma is a biopsy. A pathologist examines a small sample of tissue removed during a biopsy from an enlarged lymph node or other affected site under a microscope. In conjunction with other distinguishing characteristics, the presence of Reed-Sternberg cells validates the diagnosis of HL.

4. Blood tests, such as blood chemistry tests and complete blood counts (CBCs), are utilized to evaluate general well-being and identify irregularities, including anemia or increased concentrations of specific proteins linked to Hodgkin lymphoma.

5. Bone Marrow Biopsy: A bone marrow biopsy may be performed in certain instances to assess the potential metastasis of the lymphoma to the bone marrow, which comprises the spongy tissue located within bones.

Staging And Classification

Following the diagnosis of Hodgkin lymphoma, medical professionals employ a staging system to ascertain the disease's extent and devise suitable therapeutic interventions.

The Ann Arbor staging system, which categorizes lymphomas according to the degree of lymph node involvement and the presence of disease in other anatomical sites, is the most frequently employed for HL. These are the phases of Hodgkin lymphoma:

1. In the initial stage, the malignancy is confined to a solitary lymph node region or an organ.

2. Stage II cancer is characterized by the presence of two or more lymph node regions adjacent to the diaphragm, or by the local extension of a single lymph node region into a nearby organ or tissue.

3. Stage III: In addition to lymph node regions located on both sides of the diaphragm, the malignancy may also spread to adjacent organs or tissues.

4. In stage four, the malignancy has metastasized extensively to various organs or systems, including the liver, lungs, or bone marrow.

Hodgkin lymphoma is additionally categorized according to the attributes of the Reed-Sternberg cells, the existence or non-existence of specific proteins, and additional variables, in addition to staging. This classification facilitates prognosis and treatment decision-making.

Treatment Options

The selection of an appropriate treatment strategy for Hodgkin lymphoma is contingent upon a multitude of factors, encompassing the disease's stage, the patient's general well-being, and personal inclinations. Generally, treatment consists of a combination of therapies designed to induce remission and discourage relapse. Frequent therapeutic alternatives for Hodgkin lymphoma consist of:

1. An essential component of the treatment for Hodgkin lymphoma, chemotherapy is based on the utilization of potent medicines to eradicate cancerous cells. Chemotherapy regimens frequently consist of drug combinations and are executed in cycles spanning multiple months.

2. Radiation Therapy: To target and eradicate cancer cells, radiation therapy employs high-energy X-rays or other forms of radiation. It can be

administered singly or in conjunction with chemotherapy, specifically for Hodgkin lymphoma in its early stages or when the disease is confined to a particular region.

3. Targeted therapies are pharmaceutical interventions that selectively concentrate on particular molecules or pathways that are implicated in the progression and endurance of cancer. An illustration of targeted therapy is brentuximab vedotin, which specifically targets the CD30 protein present in Reed-Sternberg cells in numerous instances of Hodgkin lymphoma.

4. Immunotherapy: To combat cancer, immunotherapy utilizes the strength of the immune system. As an example of immunotherapy, checkpoint inhibitors (Nivolumab and Pembrolizumab) assist the immune system in identifying and eliminating cancer cells.

5. Stem Cell Transplantation: Stem cell transplantation may be considered in certain instances, especially in the case of relapsed or refractory Hodgkin lymphoma. This methodology entails the substitution of afflicted bone marrow with viable stem cells, which may originate from the patient (allogeneic transplant) or a donor (autologous transplant).

6. Clinical Trials: Certain patients diagnosed with Hodgkin lymphoma, especially those with advanced or treatment-resistant disease, may have the opportunity to participate in clinical trials. In clinical trials, novel therapeutic interventions or combinations thereof are assessed to improve patient outcomes among cancer patients.

Hodgkin lymphoma treatment options are extremely individualized, necessitating meticulous evaluation of the advantages and disadvantages of each strategy. Medical oncologists, radiation oncologists, hematologists, and other specialists comprise multidisciplinary teams of healthcare providers who collaborate to develop individualized treatment plans that are specific to the requirements and preferences of each patient.

In conclusion, Hodgkin lymphoma necessitates a comprehensive approach to both diagnosis and treatment due to its heterogeneous and complex nature. In recent years, patient outcomes have been vastly improved due to developments in the understanding of the biology of HL and the creation of novel treatment strategies; numerous individuals have achieved long-term remission or even complete recovery.

Nevertheless, continuous research endeavors are required to enhance therapeutic methodologies and maximize results for every patient impacted by this formidable malignancy.

CHAPTER THREE

The Use Of Chemotherapy

A frequent course of treatment for Hodgkin lymphoma is chemotherapy. It involves the use of medications to target swiftly dividing cells throughout the body to eliminate cancer cells. Substances used in chemotherapy may be administered subcutaneously, intravenously, or via injection. By circulating through the circulation, the medications can reach cancer cells in various regions of the body.

Chemotherapy is frequently employed as the principal therapeutic approach for patients with advanced stages of Hodgkin lymphoma or those who are at an increased risk of recurrence. The potential for its combination with additional therapeutic modalities, including immunotherapy or radiation therapy, is contingent upon the particular attributes of the malignancy and the overall well-being of the patient.

In the case of Hodgkin lymphoma, chemotherapy regimens generally comprise a combination of medications, including BEACOPP (bleomycin, etoposide, doxorubicin, cyclophosphamide, vincristine, procarbazine, and prednisone) or ABVD (doxorubicin, bleomycin, vinblastine, and dacarbazine). The selection of a treatment plan is contingent upon various considerations, including the patient's age, general health, disease stage, and the existence of concurrent medical conditions.

Chemotherapy may be efficacious in eradicating malignant cells; however, its influence on healthy cells within the body may result in adverse effects. Chemotherapy-induced adverse effects in individuals with Hodgkin lymphoma may manifest as anemia, fatigue, hair loss, and an elevated susceptibility to infection.

Although many of these adverse effects are manageable with supportive care, they frequently improve following treatment.

Radiation Treatment

In addition to radiotherapy, radiation therapy is a crucial treatment modality for Hodgkin lymphoma. The procedure entails the application of high-energy radiation to specifically target and eradicate malignant cells while mitigating harm to adjacent healthy tissue. External beam radiation therapy (EBRT) involves the utilization of a linear accelerator to administer radiation therapy externally, whereas brachytherapy involves the insertion of radioactive materials directly into or near the tumor for internal delivery.

Radiation therapy is frequently combined with chemotherapy to treat Hodgkin lymphoma, particularly in cases of early-stage disease or limited localized involvement. It can be utilized after chemotherapy to specifically target any remaining disease or as the principal treatment for patients who do not qualify for chemotherapy.

The utilization of radiation therapy for Hodgkin lymphoma is contingent upon a multitude of considerations, encompassing the disease's stage and site, the existence of specific risk factors, the patient's general well-being, and personal inclinations. By targeting specific lymph node regions or areas of voluminous disease identified through imaging studies, radiation therapy can be administered.

Fatigue, skin irritation or blisters at the site of treatment, vertigo, and long-term complications such as an increased risk of developing secondary malignancies are some of the adverse effects that may accompany radiation therapy, despite its potential for effective treatment of Hodgkin lymphoma. Several variables affect the likelihood of adverse effects occurring during radiation therapy, including the treatment site, dosage, and duration, as well as the patient's unique attributes.

The Use Of Immunotherapy

An increasingly prevalent method of treating cancer, immunotherapy utilizes the immune system to identify and eliminate malignant cells. Among specific patients diagnosed with Hodgkin lymphoma, immunotherapy medications referred to as checkpoint inhibitors have demonstrated encouraging outcomes.

Checkpoint inhibitors function by obstructing checkpoint molecules, which are proteins utilized by cancer cells to elude immune system detection. By impeding the activity of these proteins, checkpoint inhibitors can enhance the immune system's capacity to identify and eliminate malignant cells.

Under approval for the treatment of Hodgkin lymphoma, pembrolizumab is a checkpoint inhibitor that specifically targets the programmed cell death protein 1 (PD-1) pathway. In patients with relapsed or refractory Hodgkin lymphoma who have not responded to other therapies, such as stem cell transplantation and chemotherapy, pembrolizumab is effective.

When patients are unable to tolerate other treatments or have relapsed or resistant disease, immunotherapy is typically the treatment of choice. Whether utilized in isolation or conjunction with targeted agents or chemotherapy, its efficacy is contingent upon the particular attributes of the malignancy and the circumstances of the individual patient.

Although immunotherapy has demonstrated efficacy in certain patients, it is important to note that treatment resistance exists and adverse effects are possible. In addition to diarrhea, pruritus, and fatigue, checkpoint inhibitors may induce inflammation of the liver, lungs, or other organs. There are instances where these adverse effects may be severe or even fatal, necessitating the vigilant supervision and control of medical professionals.

To summarise, Hodgkin lymphoma is a lymphatic system malignancy distinguished by the existence of Reed-Sternberg cells. Chemotherapy, radiation therapy, and immunotherapy are all viable treatment modalities for Hodgkin lymphoma. The specific combination or alternative of these approaches is determined by the disease's stage, characteristics, and the patient's general health. Every one of these treatment modalities possesses unique advantages and possible adverse effects, and the selection of treatment is customized to suit the specific requirements and conditions of each patient.

CHAPTER FOUR

Cell Stem Transplantation

Hematopoietic stem cell transplantation (HSCT), alternatively referred to as stem cell transplantation, is a therapeutic approach employed to address a range of malignancies, including Hodgkin lymphoma. It entails the transplantation of healthy stem cells into diseased or damaged bone marrow (the spongy tissue found within bones). Stem cells may be obtained from a donor (allogeneic transplantation) or the patient (autologous transplantation).

Stimulatory responses to standard therapies or relapses following initial treatment are frequent circumstances in which stem cell transplantation is contemplated in the context of Hodgkin lymphoma. The transplantation procedure generally comprises the following stages:

1.	Preparation:	High-dose	chemotherapy and occasionally radiation therapy	are administered to the patient before the transplant to eliminate cancer cells and suppress the immune system, thereby preventing rejection of the transplanted cells.

2. Harvesting: Stem cells are extracted from the patient's blood or bone marrow before high-dose therapy in autologous transplantation. Allogeneic transplantation involves the procurement of stem cells from a compatible donor, who is typically identified through a matching procedure as either a close relative or an unrelated individual.

3.	Transplantation involves	a	comparable procedure to a blood transfusion: the gathered stem cells are introduced into the patient's circulation via a vein. The stem cells migrate to the bone marrow after infusion, where they initiate the production of new, healthy blood cells.

4. Recovery: The patient undergoes vigilant observation for complications, including infections, graft-versus-host disease (in the case of allogeneic transplantation), and adverse effects of the high-dose therapy, following transplantation. The full restoration of the immune system could require several weeks to months. In certain instances of Hodgkin lymphoma, stem cell transplantation may present a viable prospect for sustained remission or even complete recovery, especially among patients who are at high risk or have experienced relapse or resistance to the disease. However, it necessitates meticulous patient selection and management by a specialized medical team and entails the risk of severe complications.

Aim-Specific Therapy

A form of cancer treatment known as targeted therapy targets and inhibits particular molecules that are implicated in the development and metastasis of cancerous cells. In contrast to conventional chemotherapy, which indiscriminately targets rapidly proliferating cells, targeted therapies are engineered to selectively target cancer cells while minimizing harm to healthy cells.

Targeted therapies have emerged as potentially effective treatment options in Hodgkin lymphoma, specifically for patients who have experienced relapse following standard therapies or who are unable to tolerate intensive chemotherapy. In Hodgkin lymphoma, targeted therapy includes the administration of monoclonal antibodies, including rituximab and brentuximab vedotin.

• Brentuximab Vedotin: This monoclonal antibody-drug conjugate targets CD30, an overexpressed protein on the surface of certain non-Hodgkin lymphoma cells as well as Hodgkin lymphoma cells. Brentuximab vedotin (BVD-) inhibits the division of healthy cells while specifically targeting cancer cells with a potent chemotherapy drug via the CD30 receptor.

• Rituximab: Although its main application is the treatment of B-cell non-Hodgkin lymphomas, specific subtypes of Hodgkin lymphoma that express the CD20 protein have also demonstrated the effectiveness of rituximab. Rituximab induces an immune response that aims to eliminate neoplastic B-cells by binding to CD20, a component found on their surface.

Additional targeted therapies under investigation for Hodgkin lymphoma encompass inhibitors of signaling pathways that are implicated in the proliferation and survival of cancer cells. For instance, inhibitors of the PD-1/PD-L1 immune checkpoint pathway are among these.

Targeted therapies can provide Hodgkin lymphoma patients with potentially more efficacious and less hazardous treatment alternatives, especially when utilized in conjunction with conventional chemotherapy or other therapeutic agents. Nevertheless, the gradual emergence of resistance to targeted therapies underscores the criticality of continuous investigation into innovative therapeutic approaches.

Supportive Management And Care

Supportive care is of paramount importance in the comprehensive management of individuals afflicted with Hodgkin lymphoma, as its objectives are to mitigate symptoms, control treatment-related adverse effects, and enhance quality of life throughout the course of the disease. Possible supportive care interventions consist of:

1. Symptom Management: Hodgkin lymphoma patients may encounter distressing manifestations including fever, fatigue, pain, and vertigo, all of which have the potential to

substantially impair their overall well-being. Medication, lifestyle adjustments, and complementary therapies may be incorporated into symptom management strategies to alleviate these symptoms.

2. Nutritional Support: Patients undergoing treatment for Hodgkin lymphoma must ensure they maintain appropriate nutrition, as radiation therapy and chemotherapy can suppress appetite and cause weight loss. Dietitians may advise patients to seek nutritional support through the use of supplements to guarantee adequate intake of vital nutrients and sustain energy levels.

3. Psychosocial Support: Patients and their families may experience profound emotional and psychological repercussions upon receiving a cancer diagnosis. Psychosocial support services, such as education programs, counseling, and support groups, can provide patients with coping mechanisms for tension and anxiety and assist

them in overcoming the emotional challenges of living with Hodgkin lymphoma.

4. Fertility Preserving: Certain Hodgkin lymphoma treatments, specifically radiation therapy and chemotherapy, have the potential to impact the fertility of both males and females. Before initiating treatment, fertility preservation options, such as sperm or egg storage, may be presented to patients of reproductive age to safeguard their future reproductive capabilities.

5. Subsequent Care: Following the conclusion of treatment for Hodgkin lymphoma, patients are obligated to attend consistent follow-up consultations with their healthcare providers to assess the likelihood of disease recurrence, handle enduring treatment-related side effects, and attend to any persistent health issues. As part of the follow-up care process, physical examinations, imaging tests, and blood testing may be

performed to evaluate the response to treatment and identify early indicators of disease recurrence.

Supportive care interventions are an essential component of the multidisciplinary approach to managing Hodgkin lymphoma and are individualized for each patient.

CHAPTER FIVE

Survival And Prognosis Rates

Several variables influence the prognosis for Hodgkin lymphoma, including the disease's stage at the time of diagnosis, the presence of specific risk factors, the subtype of Hodgkin lymphoma, and the patient's response to treatment. In comparison to numerous other forms of cancer, Hodgkin lymphoma exhibits a comparatively high rate of successful remission or complete recovery for the majority of patients through the implementation of suitable therapeutic interventions.

The prognosis of Hodgkin lymphoma is frequently evaluated using the International Prognostic Score (IPS), which takes into account various factors including disease stage, age, the presence of B symptoms (night sweats, fever, weight loss), and specific blood marker levels (erythrocyte sedimentation rate and serum albumin).

Even for patients with advanced or relapsed Hodgkin lymphoma, treatment advancements such as combination chemotherapy, radiation therapy, stem cell transplantation, and targeted therapies have resulted in improved prognoses.

The overall 5-year relative survival rate for Hodgkin lymphoma is approximately 87%, as reported by the American Cancer Society. This means that approximately 87 out of every 100 individuals who are diagnosed with Hodgkin lymphoma will maintain survival for a minimum of five years following their diagnosis. Nevertheless, it is critical to bear in mind that survival rates are statistical approximations derived from sizable cohorts of patients and might not precisely portend the prognosis of an individual.

The advanced stage at the time of diagnosis, advanced age, specific subtypes of Hodgkin lymphoma (e.g., nodular lymphocyte-predominant Hodgkin lymphoma), and initial treatment failure without achieving complete remission are all associated with an unfavorable prognosis in this disease.

In general, continuous investigation into the biological mechanisms underlying Hodgkin lymphoma, coupled with the advancement of innovative therapeutic strategies, serves to elevate patient prognoses and deepen our comprehension of this intricate ailment.

Preventive Measures

Due to the intricate interplay of genetic, environmental, and immunological factors that contribute to its development, Hodgkin lymphoma prevention is difficult. Some strategies, however, may aid in mitigating the risk or postponing its initiation:

1. Adhering to a healthy lifestyle, which entails consuming a well-balanced diet abundant in whole cereals, fruits, and vegetables, and engaging in consistent physical activity, could potentially mitigate the likelihood of developing Hodgkin lymphoma.

2. It is advisable to abstain from tobacco and alcohol usage, as these substances have been linked to an elevated likelihood of developing Hodgkin lymphoma. Reducing or avoiding contact with these substances could potentially mitigate the associated risk.

3. Preventing Infections: Specific viral infections, including Epstein-Barr virus (EBV), have been associated with an elevated likelihood of developing Hodgkin lymphoma. Implementing preventive measures, such as maintaining proper

hygiene, avoiding direct contact with individuals who are infected with infectious mononucleosis (EBV-caused strains), and receiving vaccinations against EBV and other viruses, can potentially mitigate the risk.

4. Reducing exposure to potential carcinogens in the workplace or environment, including but not limited to industrial chemicals, pesticides, and solvents, may additionally aid in mitigating the likelihood of developing Hodgkin lymphoma.

5. Consistent medical examinations—early detection of Hodgkin lymphoma could potentially enhance treatment efficacy. To detect any early signs or symptoms, individuals with a family history of lymphoma or other malignancies should endure routine medical screenings and examinations.

Although these approaches might aid in mitigating the likelihood of developing Hodgkin lymphoma, it is critical to emphasize that complete prevention is not feasible due to the elusive etiology of this malignancy.

Recent Developments And Research

Considerable advancements in knowledge have been achieved regarding Hodgkin lymphoma, resulting in enhanced methods of diagnosis, treatment alternatives, and overall prognoses. The following are notable sectors of research and development:

1. Inhibitors of immune checkpoints and monoclonal antibodies are examples of targeted therapies that have significantly transformed the management of Hodgkin lymphoma. Particularly designed to inhibit specific molecules or pathways implicated in the progression and growth of cancer, these

medications produce fewer adverse effects than conventional chemotherapy.

2. Immunotherapy: By enhancing the body's immune response against cancer cells, immunotherapy, specifically immune checkpoint inhibitors such as pembrolizumab and nivolumab, has demonstrated encouraging outcomes in the treatment of relapsed or refractory Hodgkin lymphoma.

3. The utilization of genomic sequencing technologies has facilitated the development of precision medicine by allowing scientists to discern particular genetic mutations or biomarkers that are linked to Hodgkin lymphoma. This data facilitates individualized treatment strategies that are specifically designed to address the unique attributes of every patient's illness.

4. Stem Cell Transplantation: For eligible patients with Hodgkin lymphoma, high-dose chemotherapy

followed by autologous stem cell transplantation continues to be the standard treatment option. Continual investigations strive to enhance transplant protocols, diminish complications, and augment long-term results.

5. Novel Therapeutic Targets: In an ongoing effort to surmount resistance and increase overall survival rates, researchers are continuously investigating new therapeutic targets and treatment modalities for Hodgkin lymphoma, including small molecule inhibitors, epigenetic modifiers, and novel immunotherapies.

Notwithstanding these advancements, substantial concerns persist regarding the management of Hodgkin lymphoma, including treatment resistance, disease relapse, and long-term adverse effects. These issues underscore the criticality of continuous research and innovation in this domain.

Coping With Hodgkin Lymphoma In Daily Life

A Hodgkin's lymphoma diagnosis can be debilitating, but many individuals can lead fulfilling lives with the assistance of suitable lifestyle modifications, emotional support, and medical treatment. The following are some coping mechanisms for Hodgkin lymphoma:

1. Adherence to Treatment: It is critical to comply with the treatment regimen as prescribed by your healthcare team. This entails attending all scheduled appointments, taking prescribed medications, and enduring any required testing or procedures.

2. A healthful lifestyle can contribute to the preservation of one's general well-being throughout and following treatment. This consists of adhering to a healthcare provider-recommended physical activity regimen, maintaining a well-

balanced diet, ensuring adequate rest, and avoiding hazardous substances such as tobacco and excessive alcohol consumption.

3. The experience of managing a cancer diagnosis can present significant emotional difficulties. To navigate the emotional challenges associated with living with Hodgkin lymphoma, it is advisable to seek assistance from mental health professionals, companions, family members, or support groups.

4. Side Effect Management: Hodgkin lymphoma treatment may induce adverse effects including fatigue, vertigo, hair loss, and alterations in appetite. Discuss with your healthcare team methods for enhancing your quality of life while undergoing treatment and managing these adverse effects.

5. Consistent follow-up appointments with your healthcare provider are imperative following treatment completion. These appointments serve

the purpose of monitoring your health, promptly identifying any indications of recurrence or complications, and attending to any persistent concerns or requirements.

6. One should participate in self-care practices that foster relaxation, alleviate tension, and involve outdoor time, yoga, meditation, or other similar activities. It is crucial to prioritize one's physical and emotional well-being while managing the challenges of living with Hodgkin lymphoma.

You can maintain a positive outlook on life and effectively manage Hodgkin lymphoma by engaging in active treatment participation, seeking support when necessary, and prioritizing self-care. Remember that each individual's path is distinct and that it is acceptable to seek assistance at any point.

Summary

In summary, Hodgkin lymphoma continues to be a substantial issue within the field of oncology, despite its relatively low incidence. This extensive synopsis has illuminated multiple facets of the ailment, including its epidemiological profile, causal factors, clinical manifestations, diagnostic methods, and therapeutic approaches.

A comprehensive comprehension of the unique subtypes, specifically classical Hodgkin lymphoma (cHL) and nodular lymphocyte-predominant Hodgkin lymphoma (NLPHL), is critical for developing individualized treatment approaches. Diagnostic precision has been significantly transformed by developments in imaging techniques, including PET-CT scans, which enable precise staging and monitoring of treatment response.

With the incorporation of immunotherapy, radiation therapy, chemotherapy, and other modalities into treatment, patient outcomes have improved substantially over time. The introduction of targeted therapies and immunomodulatory agents has opened up novel approaches to the management of cases that are resistant or relapsed, resulting in increased rates of survival and improved quality of life.

Furthermore, current research initiatives dedicated to elucidating the molecular mechanisms that underlie the pathogenesis of Hodgkin lymphoma offer the potential for the development of future treatment regimens that are more individualized and efficacious. Nevertheless, obstacles endure, such as the potential for permanent complications associated with treatment and the imperative for diligent monitoring to identify possible relapses.

Fundamentally, despite significant advancements in the comprehension and control of Hodgkin lymphoma, ongoing research endeavors, and collaborative undertakings are indispensable for the ultimate enhancement of therapeutic strategies and the improvement of patient prognoses.

THE END